# YOGA FOR BEGINNERS

VIJAY PATIDAR

Made with ♥ on the Notion Press Platform
www.notionpress.com

# Contents

# Preface

Yoga is an ancient practice that has been around for thousands of years. Originating in India, it is a holistic practice that incorporates physical postures (asanas), breathing techniques (pranayama), meditation, and philosophy. Yoga is not just a form of exercise; it is a way of life that can improve both the mind and body.

The word "yoga" comes from the Sanskrit word "yuj" which means "to unite or join". In yoga, the focus is on uniting the mind, body, and breath. This is achieved through the practice of physical postures, breathing techniques, and meditation.

Yoga has been around for over 5,000 years and has evolved over time. The earliest form of yoga was known as "Vedic yoga" and it was mainly used for spiritual practices and rituals. Later on, Patanjali, an Indian sage, compiled the Yoga Sutras, which is considered the foundation of classical yoga. The Yoga Sutras outline the 8 limbs of yoga, which includes physical postures, breathing techniques, and meditation.

Yoga is beneficial for both the mind and body. Physically, it can help increase flexibility, strength, and balance. It can also help with weight loss and improve overall cardiovascular health. Mentally, yoga can help reduce stress, anxiety, and depression. It can also improve focus and concentration.

Yoga is a low-impact form of exercise, making it suitable for people of all ages and fitness levels. It is important to start with basic poses and gradually work your way up to more advanced poses. It is also important to listen to your body and not push yourself too hard.

In this eBook, we will be discussing the basics of yoga and how to start a yoga practice as a beginner. We will delve into the physical postures, breathing techniques, and meditation that make up yoga. We will also explore the philosophy of yoga and how it can enhance your practice.

Remember, yoga is a practice and it takes time to see progress. Be patient with yourself and enjoy the journey

**History of yoga**

The history of yoga can be traced back over 5,000 years to ancient India, where it was initially developed as a spiritual practice. The earliest form of yoga, known as "Vedic yoga," was mainly used for spiritual practices and rituals. The Vedas, which are ancient Hindu texts, contain references to yoga practices and philosophy.

Over time, yoga evolved and developed into different forms. The Yoga Sutras, written by the Indian sage Patanjali, is considered the foundation of classical yoga. The Yoga Sutras outline the 8 limbs of yoga, which includes physical postures, breathing techniques, and meditation. This form of yoga is known as Raja yoga or "royal yoga" and is considered the path of self-control and discipline.

In addition to Raja yoga, there are several other forms of yoga that have developed over time, including:

Hatha yoga: This form of yoga emphasizes the physical practice of yoga and is focused on developing strength, flexibility, and balance.

Bhakti yoga: This form of yoga is focused on devotion and the cultivation of love and devotion towards a personal deity.

Karma yoga: This form of yoga is focused on selfless service and the performance of actions without attachment to the results.

Jnana yoga: This form of yoga is focused on the pursuit of knowledge and self-realization through study and contemplation.

In the $20^{th}$ century, yoga began to gain popularity in the West. Many Westerners were introduced to yoga through the teachings of Indian gurus who came to the West to share their knowledge. In the 1960s and 1970s, yoga experienced a surge in popularity in the United States and Europe, and it has continued to grow in popularity in the years since. Today, yoga is widely recognized as a form of exercise and a complementary therapy for various health conditions.

It is important to note that the history of yoga is vast and complex, and this is just a brief overview of the evolution of yoga over time. There are many different styles, traditions, and lineages of yoga that have developed over the centuries, each with its own unique approach to the practice.

**Benefits of yoga**

Yoga is a practice that can benefit both the mind and body. Some of the most well-known benefits of yoga include:

Improves flexibility: Yoga involves a series of physical postures, or asanas, that help to stretch and strengthen the muscles. Regular practice can increase flexibility and range of motion in the joints.

Builds strength: Yoga poses work the muscles, building strength and endurance. Yoga also help in balance, it can also help improve balance, stability, and coordination.

Improves cardiovascular health: Yoga breathing exercises, known as pranayama, can help to lower blood pressure and improve circulation.

Reduces stress and anxiety: Yoga's focus on breathing and meditation can help to reduce stress and anxiety. The physical practice of yoga can also help to release tension from the body.

Improves sleep: Yoga can help to relax the body and mind, making it easier to fall asleep and stay asleep.

Improves mental health: Yoga can help to improve focus, concentration and memory. The practice of yoga and meditation can also help to reduce symptoms of depression and anxiety.

Enhances spiritual growth: Yoga encourages self-reflection and self-awareness, which can lead to spiritual growth and a deeper understanding of oneself.

It's important to note that although the benefits of yoga are well-documented, it's always best to consult with a healthcare professional before starting any new exercise program, particularly if you have any health conditions.

CHAPTER ONE

# Yoga for the Body

Yoga for the Body involves the practice of physical postures, or asanas, that help to stretch and strengthen the muscles. The practice of yoga can improve flexibility, strength, balance, and overall physical health.

Basic yoga poses for beginners include:

Mountain Pose (Tadasana): This is a standing pose that helps to improve posture and balance.

Downward-Facing Dog (Adho Mukha Svanasana): This is an inverted pose that helps to stretch the entire body.

Child's Pose (Balasana): This is a resting pose that can help to release tension in the back and shoulders.

Cobra Pose (Bhujangasana): This is a gentle backbend that can help to strengthen the spine.

Warrior Pose (Virabhadrasana): This is a standing pose that can help to strengthen the legs and core.

It is important to start with basic poses and gradually work your way up to more advanced poses. It is also important to listen to your body and not push yourself too hard. It is important to focus on proper alignment and form, as well as using modifications and variations to accommodate different fitness levels.

It is always recommended to take a class with a qualified yoga teacher in the beginning, to learn the proper form and alignment, and to avoid injury. As you become more comfortable with the practice, you can then start to incorporate a yoga practice into your daily routine.

Additionally, Yoga for the body can be modified for different populations such as pregnant women, seniors, and children. There are also specific styles of yoga like restorative yoga, yin yoga, and power yoga that focus on certain aspects of physical fitness and well-being.

In summary, yoga for the body is a holistic practice that can improve flexibility, strength, balance and overall physical health. It's important to start with basic poses, focus on proper alignment and form, and listen to your body. It is always recommended to take a class with a qualified yoga teacher in the beginning, to learn the proper form and alignment, and to avoid injury.

**Physical postures (asanas)**

Physical postures, or asanas, are one of the key components of yoga practice. These postures are designed to stretch and strengthen the muscles, while also improving flexibility, balance, and overall physical health.

There are many different types of asanas, each with its own unique benefits. Some of the most common asanas include:

Standing poses: These poses are designed to improve posture, balance, and core strength. Examples include Tadasana (Mountain Pose), Virabhadrasana (Warrior Pose), and Trikonasana (Triangle Pose).

Sitting poses: These poses are designed to improve flexibility in the hips and legs. Examples include Padmasana (Lotus Pose), Sukhasana (Easy Pose), and Virasana (Hero Pose).

Inverted poses: These poses are designed to improve circulation, energize the body, and calm the mind. Examples include Adho Mukha Svanasana (Downward-Facing Dog), Sirsasana (Headstand), and Sarvangasana (Shoulder Stand).

Backbends: These poses are designed to open the chest, improve breathing, and increase flexibility in the spine. Examples include Bhujangasana (Cobra Pose), Urdhva Mukha Svanasana (Upward-Facing Dog), and Dhanurasana (Bow Pose).

Forward bends: These poses are designed to stretch the back and legs and calm the mind. Examples include Paschimottanasana (Seated Forward Bend), Uttanasana (Standing Forward Bend), and Janu Sirsasana (Head-to-Knee Pose).

It is important to remember that asanas should be practiced with proper alignment and form to avoid injury. It's also important to listen to your body and not push yourself too hard. Some people may not be able to perform certain asanas due to physical limitations, and modifications can be made to accommodate these limitations.

It's always recommended to take a class with a qualified yoga teacher to learn proper alignment and form and to avoid injury. As you become more comfortable with the practice, you can then start to incorporate a yoga practice into your daily routine, and can explore different styles of yoga that focus on certain aspects of physical fitness and well-being.

**Basic yoga poses for beginners**

Basic yoga poses for beginners are designed to be easy to perform, and are often used as a starting point for a yoga practice. These poses can help to improve flexibility, strength, and balance, and can be modified to accommodate different fitness levels. Here are some examples of basic yoga poses for beginners:

Tadasana (Mountain Pose): This is a standing pose that helps to improve posture and balance. To perform Tadasana, stand with your feet together and your arms at your sides. Draw your shoulders back and engage your core.

Adho Mukha Svanasana (Downward Facing Dog): This is an inverted pose that helps to stretch the entire body. To perform Adho Mukha Svanasana, start on your hands and knees. Lift your hips up and back, straightening your arms and legs.

Balasana (Child's Pose): This is a resting pose that can help to release tension in the back and shoulders. To perform Balasana, start on your hands and knees. Lower your hips back to your heels and stretch your arms out in front of you.

Bhujangasana (Cobra Pose): This is a gentle backbend that can help to strengthen the spine. To perform Bhujangasana, start on your stomach with your hands under your shoulders. Slowly lift your chest off the ground, keeping your elbows close to your body.

Virabhadrasana (Warrior Pose): This is a standing pose that can help to strengthen the legs and core. To perform Virabhadrasana, start in Tadasana. Step one foot back, and bend the front knee. Stretch your arms out to the side, and look forward.

These are just a few examples of basic yoga poses for beginners. It's always recommended to take a class with a qualified yoga teacher to learn proper alignment and form, and to avoid injury. As you become more comfortable with the practice, you can then start to incorporate a yoga practice into your daily routine and explore different styles of yoga that focus on certain aspects of physical fitness and well-being.

**Importance of alignment and proper form**

The importance of alignment and proper form in yoga practice cannot be overstated. Proper alignment and form ensure that the poses are being performed safely and effectively, reducing the risk of injury and maximizing the benefits of the practice.

Proper alignment means positioning the body in a way that is safe and efficient for the joints and muscles. This includes aligning the bones and joints in a neutral position, and engaging the appropriate muscles to support the pose. Proper alignment also helps to prevent over-stretching or straining of the muscles, which can lead to injury.

Proper form refers to the precise execution of the movement or pose. This includes moving in and out of the pose with control, and maintaining the appropriate muscle engagement throughout the pose. Proper form also helps to prevent over-stretching or straining of the muscles, and can help to improve the effectiveness of the pose.

When starting a yoga practice, it is important to learn the proper alignment and form of the poses from a qualified yoga teacher. As you become more familiar with the practice, you can then begin to incorporate these principles into your home practice.

Proper alignment and form also help to create a meditative state, allowing the mind and body to work together in harmony. This leads to a deeper and more fulfilling yoga practice that can be beneficial for both the body and mind.

In summary, proper alignment and form in yoga practice is important for safety and effectiveness. It reduces the risk of injury and maximizes the benefits of the practice. It is always recommended to learn proper alignment and form from a qualified yoga teacher.

**Modifications and variations for different fitness levels for Yoga**

Modifications and variations for different fitness levels are important for making yoga accessible and safe for everyone. These adjustments can help to accommodate different physical abilities and can make the practice more comfortable and beneficial for the individual.

Here are a few examples of modifications and variations for different fitness levels:

For beginners or those with limited flexibility: Use props such as blocks or blankets to assist with balance and alignment in poses. Reduce the range of motion in certain poses, or use a wall or chair for support.

For people with injuries or chronic pain: Avoid poses that put pressure on the injured area, and instead focus on poses that can help to strengthen the surrounding muscles. Use props such as blocks or straps to assist with balance and alignment in poses.

For people who are pregnant: Avoid poses that put pressure on the abdomen, such as backbends or twists. Instead, focus on poses that can help to strengthen the legs and core, such as downward-facing dog or warrior.

For people who are older: Avoid poses that put pressure on the joints, such as forward bends or twists. Instead, focus on poses that can help to improve balance and flexibility, such as mountain pose or tree pose.

It's important to remember that everyone's body is different, and what might be a modification for one person may not be for another. It's always recommended to consult with a qualified yoga teacher to determine the best modifications and variations for your individual needs and fitness level.

In summary, modifications and variations for different fitness levels are important for making yoga accessible and safe for everyone. They can help to accommodate different physical abilities and make the practice more comfortable and beneficial for the individual. It's always recommended to consult with a qualified yoga teacher to determine the best modifications and variations for your individual needs and fitness level.

CHAPTER TWO

# Yoga for the Breath

Yoga for the breath, also known as pranayama, is an essential component of yoga practice. It involves the use of specific breathing techniques to control the flow of prana, or vital energy, throughout the body.

Pranayama can help to improve respiratory function, increase lung capacity, and reduce stress and anxiety. It also has a direct impact on the nervous system, helping to balance the sympathetic and parasympathetic systems, which can lead to a reduction in stress and a sense of calmness and well-being.

Here are a few examples of basic pranayama techniques for beginners:

Ujjayi breath: This breath is also known as "victorious breath," and is characterized by a slight constriction of the throat, creating a soft sound as the breath is inhaled and exhaled. This breath helps to calm the mind, and is often used during yoga practice.

Nadi Shodhana (Alternate Nostril Breathing): This breath helps to balance the left and right side of the brain and body. It's done by closing one nostril and inhaling and exhaling through the other and then switching.

Kapalabhati (Skull-Shining Breath): This breath is a powerful and energizing breath that helps to clear the lungs and sinuses. It's done by forcefully exhaling and then passively inhaling.

Bhramari (Humming Bee Breath): This breath is a calming breath that is done by making a humming sound as you exhale. It helps to release tension in the head and neck, and can be helpful for reducing stress and anxiety.

It's important to note that, as with any yoga practice, it's always recommended to learn the proper technique for pranayama from a qualified yoga teacher, especially if you have any medical conditions related to breathing.

In summary, Yoga for the breath, also known as pranayama, is an essential component of yoga practice. It involves the use of specific breathing techniques to control the flow of prana, or vital energy, throughout the body.

**Overview of pranayama (yoga breathing techniques)**

Pranayama, or yoga breathing techniques, is an essential component of yoga practice. It involves the use of specific breathing techniques to control the flow of prana, or vital energy, throughout the body. Pranayama can help to improve respiratory function, increase lung capacity, and reduce stress and anxiety. It also has a direct impact on the nervous system, helping to balance the sympathetic and parasympathetic systems, which can lead to a reduction in stress and a sense of calmness and well-being.

There are many different types of pranayama, each with its own unique benefits. Some of the most well-known pranayama techniques include:

Ujjayi breath: Also known as "Victorious breath," this breath is characterized by a slight constriction of the throat, creating a soft sound as the breath is inhaled and exhaled. This breath helps to calm the mind and is often used during yoga practice.

Nadi Shodhana (Alternate Nostril Breathing): This breath helps to balance the left and right side of the brain and body. It's done by closing one nostril and inhaling and exhaling through the other and then switching.

Kapalabhati (Skull-Shining Breath): This breath is a powerful and energizing breath that helps to clear the lungs and sinuses. It's done by forcefully exhaling and then passively inhaling.

Bhramari (Humming Bee Breath): This breath is a calming breath that is done by making a humming sound as you exhale. It helps to release tension in the head and neck, and can be helpful for reducing stress and anxiety.

Sitali breath: This cooling breath is done by inhaling through a curled tongue and exhaling through the nose. It helps to reduce heat in the body and mind, and can be helpful for reducing stress and anxiety.

Bhastrika breath: This breath is done by rapidly inhaling and exh

**Common breathing techniques for beginners**

There are many different pranayama techniques, some of which can be quite advanced and require a certain level of experience and skill. However, for beginners, there are several breathing techniques that are considered to be more accessible and easier to learn. Here are a few examples of common breathing techniques for beginners:

Diaphragmatic breathing: Also known as "belly breathing," this technique involves breathing deeply into the diaphragm, rather than shallowly into the chest. To practice diaphragmatic breathing, lie down on your back, place one hand on your chest and the other on your belly. As you inhale, allow your belly to rise, and as you exhale, allow your belly to fall.

Ujjayi breath: This breath is also known as "victorious breath," and is characterized by a slight constriction of the throat, creating a soft sound as the breath is inhaled and exhaled. To practice Ujjayi breath, inhale and exhale through the nose, constricting the back of the throat slightly as you exhale.

Nadi Shodhana (Alternate Nostril Breathing): This breath helps to balance the left and right side of the brain and body. To practice Nadi Shodhana, sit in a comfortable position and use your right thumb to close your right nostril. Inhale through your left nostril, then use your ring finger to close your left nostril and exhale through your right nostril.

Box breathing: This technique is also called "square breathing" and can be helpful for stress and anxiety. To practice box breathing, inhale for a count of 4, hold for a count of 4, exhale for a count of 4, and hold for a count of 4 before starting again.

It’s important to note that for all the breathing techniques, it’s important to breathe in a comfortable, relaxed manner and never force the breath. It’s always recommended to learn these breathing techniques from a qualified yoga teacher to ensure proper technique and to avoid injury.

**Importance of breath control in yoga practice**

Breath control, or pranayama, plays a crucial role in yoga practice. The breath is considered to be the link between the mind and body, and the control of the breath can have a direct impact on both physical and mental well-being.

Here are a few ways in which breath control is important in yoga practice:

Increases lung capacity: Pranayama techniques can help to increase lung capacity, which can lead to better oxygenation of the body’s cells and tissues. This can help to improve overall physical health, as well as mental clarity and focus.

Reduces stress and anxiety: Pranayama techniques can help to activate the parasympathetic nervous system, which can lead to a reduction in stress and anxiety. Slow, deep breathing can also help to calm the mind and reduce feelings of anxiety.

Improves concentration and focus: Pranayama techniques can help to improve concentration and focus by training the mind to focus on the breath. This can be particularly helpful during meditation and asana practice.

Enhances physical practice: Pranayama can help to increase energy levels, improve respiratory function and increase lung capacity, which can enhance the physical practice of yoga.

Enhances spiritual practice: Pranayama can help to purify the nadis (energy channels) and chakras (energy centers) in the body, which can lead to a deeper spiritual

CHAPTER THREE

# Yoga for the Mind

Yoga for the mind, also known as yoga for the mental and emotional well-being, is an important aspect of yoga practice. Yoga has been shown to have a positive impact on mental health, and can help to improve mood, reduce stress, and increase feelings of well-being.

Here are a few ways in which yoga can benefit the mind:

Reduces stress and anxiety: Yoga can help to activate the parasympathetic nervous system, which can lead to a reduction in stress and anxiety. Mindful breathing, meditation, and certain asanas (yoga poses) can also help to calm the mind and reduce feelings of anxiety.

Improves mood: Yoga has been shown to increase the production of certain neurotransmitters, such as serotonin and dopamine, which can lead to improvements in mood.

Increases self-awareness: Yoga can help to increase self-awareness by bringing attention to the present moment. This can be particularly beneficial for individuals who struggle with negative thoughts and emotions.

Enhances cognitive function: Yoga can improve cognitive function by increasing attention and focus. It can also help to improve memory and learning.

Improves sleep: Yoga can help to improve sleep by reducing feelings of stress and anxiety, which are common causes of insomnia.

Incorporating a regular yoga practice into daily life can provide numerous benefits for both the body and mind. Yoga can be especially beneficial for those experiencing stress, anxiety, and depression, but it can also be beneficial for anyone looking to improve their overall well-being. It's always recommended to consult with a qualified yoga teacher to determine the best approach for your individual needs and goals.

**Overview of meditation in yoga**

Meditation is an integral part of yoga practice. It involves the use of techniques, such as focused attention, to bring about a heightened state of awareness and inner calm.

There are many different types of meditation, each with its own unique benefits. Some of the most well-known meditation techniques in yoga include:

Mindfulness meditation: This type of meditation involves paying attention to the present moment, without judgment. It can help to increase self-awareness and reduce stress and anxiety.

Transcendental meditation: This type of meditation involves the use of a mantra, or word or phrase, to focus the mind and bring about a state of deep relaxation.

Yoga nidra: Also known as "yogic sleep," this meditation technique involves lying down in a comfortable position and guiding the mind through a series of visualizations and body scans. It can help to reduce stress and improve sleep.

Chakra meditation: This type of meditation focuses on the seven chakras, or energy centers, in the body. It can help to balance and align the chakras, leading to a sense of well-being and inner peace.

Loving-kindness meditation: Also known as "metta" meditation, this type of meditation involves focusing on feelings of love and kindness towards oneself and others. It can help to increase feelings of compassion and empathy.

It's important to note that while meditation can be beneficial for many people, it's not suitable for everyone. It's always recommended to consult with a qualified yoga teacher or healthcare professional before starting a meditation practice, especially if you have a history of mental health issues.

In summary, Meditation is an integral part of yoga practice. It involves the use of techniques, such as focused attention, to bring about a heightened state of awareness and inner calm. There are many different types of meditation, each with its own unique benefits, and can be beneficial for many people, but it's not suitable for everyone. It's always recommended to consult with a qualified yoga teacher or healthcare professional before starting a meditation practice.

**Simple meditation techniques for beginners**

Meditation can seem intimidating for beginners, but there are many simple techniques that can be easily incorporated into daily life. Here are a few examples of simple meditation techniques for beginners:

Breath awareness: Sit or lie down in a comfortable position and simply focus your attention on your breath. Notice the sensation of the breath as it enters and exits your nose or mouth. If your mind wanders, gently guide it back to the breath.

Body scan: Lie down in a comfortable position and bring your attention to different parts of your body, starting from your toes and working your way up to the crown of your head. Notice any sensations, such as tension or relaxation, and mentally release any tension you find.

Guided meditation: This can be done by listening to a recorded meditation or following along with a teacher or app. Guided meditations usually involve listening to someone's voice giving you instructions and prompts, which can be helpful for keeping the mind focused.

Loving-kindness meditation: Sit in a comfortable position and repeat phrases such as "may I be happy, may I be healthy, may I be at peace" to yourself. Then, extend these phrases to loved ones, acquaintances, and eventually, to all beings.

Yoga Nidra: This meditation technique involves lying down in a comfortable position and guiding the mind through a series of visualizations and body scans. It can help to reduce stress and improve sleep.

It's important to note that meditation is a practice, and it takes time and patience to develop the skill. It's always recommended to start with shorter meditation sessions and gradually increase the time as you become more comfortable with the practice.

In summary, there are many simple meditation techniques for beginners, such as breath awareness, body scan, guided meditation, loving-kindness meditation, and Yoga Nidra. It's important to start with shorter meditation sessions and gradually increase the time as you become more comfortable with the practice. It's always recommended to consult with a qualified yoga teacher or healthcare professional before starting a meditation practice.

**How meditation can improve mental health and well-being**

Meditation has been shown to have a positive impact on mental health and well-being. It can reduce stress, anxiety, and depression, as well as improve focus, concentration, and self-awareness. Additionally, meditation can help with emotional regulation, which is the ability to manage one's emotions in a healthy way. This can lead to better relationships and improved overall quality of life. Regular practice of meditation can also improve sleep, reduce inflammation, and even change the structure of the brain in positive ways.

CHAPTER FOUR

# Building Your Yoga Practice

Building a yoga practice involves consistently setting aside time to practice, being open to learning and trying new things, and listening to your body's needs. Here are a few tips to help you get started:

Start with a beginner class or tutorial. This will give you a solid foundation in the basics of yoga and help you understand the proper alignment and form for different poses.

Set a regular practice schedule. Whether it's once a week or every day, make a commitment to practicing at the same time each day.

Listen to your body. Yoga is not a competition, and it's important to honor your body's limitations. If a pose doesn't feel right, modify it or come out of it completely.

Be consistent. The more you practice, the more you'll see progress and the more you'll enjoy your practice.

Find a teacher or class that resonates with you. A good teacher can provide guidance, modifications, and inspiration to help you deepen your practice.

Be patient with yourself. Remember that yoga is a journey, not a destination. It takes time to see progress and to learn new poses and techniques.

Remember to breathe. Breath is the foundation of yoga practice and it helps you to stay present, focused and calm.

Keep an open mind. Yoga is a practice of self-discovery and growth, be open to trying new things and learning from your experiences.

**Finding a qualified yoga teacher**

Finding a qualified yoga teacher can be an important step in building a safe and effective yoga practice. Here are a few tips to help you find a teacher who is right for you:

Look for a teacher with a recognized yoga certification. Many reputable yoga teacher training programs require their graduates to meet certain standards of education and experience before they can be certified.

Check for insurance and liability coverage. A qualified teacher should be insured in case of injury or accidents during class.

Look for a teacher who offers modifications and adjustments. A good teacher should be able to provide modifications and adjustments for students with injuries or special needs.

Check the teacher's reviews and testimonials. Many teachers have a website or social media page with reviews from students.

Visit a class or take a trial lesson. This will give you a sense of the teacher's style and level of instruction, and will help you decide if the teacher is a good fit for you.

Ask for recommendations from friends or other yogis in your community. Word of mouth can be a powerful tool for finding a qualified teacher.

Check if the teacher is registered with Yoga Alliance. Yoga Alliance is a non-profit organization that sets standards for yoga teacher training and certifications.

Look for a teacher who has continuing education and training. A teacher who continues to learn and evolve will be able to provide a more varied and dynamic practice.

**Creating a home yoga practice**

Creating a home yoga practice can be a great way to make yoga a regular part of your daily routine. Here are a few tips to help you get started:

Set aside a specific time and place for your practice. Having a dedicated space for yoga, whether it's a corner of a room or a specific mat, can help establish a regular practice.

Make a plan. Decide what you want to focus on during your practice and choose poses and sequences that align with your goals.

Use online resources. There are many online yoga classes, tutorials, and videos that can guide you through a practice.

Use props. Yoga props such as blocks, straps, and blankets can help you safely and comfortably modify poses.

Be consistent. Make a commitment to practice at the same time every day, and make it a non-negotiable part of your daily routine.

Remember to breathe. Breath is the foundation of yoga practice and it helps you to stay present, focused and calm.

Listen to your body. Yoga is not a competition, and it's important to honor your body's limitations. If a pose doesn't feel right, modify it or come out of it completely.

Have an open mind. A home practice is a great opportunity to explore new poses, sequences and styles of yoga.

Create a comfortable environment. Make sure your practice space is quiet, well-ventilated and at a comfortable temperature.

Remember to end your practice with a relaxation or meditation. This will help you to integrate the benefits of your practice and to end in a peaceful state of mind.

**Setting goals and tracking progress**

Setting goals and tracking progress can be an effective way to stay motivated and focused on your yoga practice. Here are a few tips to help you set and track your goals:

Be specific and measurable. Instead of setting a general goal like "improve flexibility," set a specific goal like "able to touch toes with straight legs in forward fold within 3 months".

Set achievable goals. Make sure your goals are realistic and attainable, given your current level of experience and fitness.

Set a deadline. Giving yourself a deadline for achieving your goal can help you stay focused and motivated.

Create a plan. Break your goal down into smaller, manageable steps and create a plan for achieving each step.

Track your progress. Keep a journal or use an app to track your progress and monitor your progress over time.

Reflect on your progress. Take time to reflect on your progress regularly, and adjust your plan as needed to stay on track.

Celebrate your achievements. Recognize and celebrate your accomplishments, no matter how small they may seem.

Be flexible. Remember that your goals may change as you progress in your practice, and be open to adjusting them as needed.

Take progress photos. Taking progress photos can be a great way to see your progress in a more visual way.

Revisit your goals. Every few months, take a step back and reassess your goals to ensure they are still in line with what you want to achieve.

**Importance of patience and consistency**

Patience and consistency are important for a yoga practice for several reasons:

Patience allows you to listen to your body and honor its limitations. Yoga is not a competition and it's important to work within your own capabilities and not push yourself too hard.

Consistency helps to establish a regular practice. The more you practice, the more you'll see progress and the more you'll enjoy your practice.

Both patience and consistency allow for a deeper understanding of the poses. With time and practice, you can learn to explore the subtler aspects of a pose, such as alignment and breath.

Consistency can help to prevent injury. By practicing regularly, you are able to build strength and flexibility gradually, reducing the risk of injury.

Patience allows you to approach your practice with a non-judgmental attitude. It encourages you to let go of expectations and to focus on the present moment.

Consistency can help to develop focus and concentration. By practicing regularly, you'll be able to develop the ability to stay focused and centered during your practice.

Patience allows you to be open to learning and trying new things. It encourages you to be open to new poses and styles of yoga, and to explore new ways of moving.

Consistency allows you to see progress in your practice. Regular practice can help you to see progress in your flexibility, strength and balance, and to understand the benefits of yoga over time.

Patience and consistency create a sense of discipline, which can be beneficial in other areas of your life.

Yoga is not just a physical practice but also a mental one, Consistency and patience will help you to develop the ability to stay calm and centered in difficult situations, both on and off the mat.

CHAPTER FIVE

# Yoga Philosophy

Yoga is a practice that originated in ancient India and is rooted in the belief that the mind, body, and spirit are interconnected. The philosophy of yoga is vast and complex, but some of its key principles include:

The practice of yoga aims to unite the individual self (jivatma) with the universal self (paramatma)

The ultimate goal of yoga is to achieve a state of enlightenment or liberation (moksha)

The path to enlightenment is through self-discipline, self-study, and devotion to the divine.

Yoga teaches the importance of ethical principles, such as non-violence, honesty, and non-stealing, as well as non-attachment and equanimity in the face of life's challenges.

The practice of yoga includes the use of physical postures (asanas), breath control (pranayama), and meditation (dhyana) as a means of purifying the body and mind, and promoting physical and mental well-being.

Yoga also encompasses the principles of the 8 limbs of yoga which are: Yama (moral guidelines), Niyama (self-discipline), Asana (postures), Pranayama (breathing techniques), Pratyahara (sense withdrawal), Dharana (concentration), Dhyana (meditation), and Samadhi (state of enlightenment)

Yoga encourages the development of a healthy and balanced lifestyle, with emphasis on proper diet and the use of natural remedies.

The ultimate goal of yoga is to cultivate a state of inner peace, contentment, and self-realization.

Yoga is not just a physical practice, but also a spiritual one. It aims to bring balance, harmony and transcendence to the body, mind, and spirit.

Yoga is an individual practice, and each person's journey is unique, but the ultimate goal is the same: to achieve a state of inner peace and enlightenment.

**Overview of yoga philosophy**

Yoga philosophy is a collection of beliefs and practices that have evolved over thousands of years in ancient India. It is based on the belief that the body, mind, and spirit are interconnected and that the ultimate goal of yoga is to achieve a state of enlightenment or liberation (moksha).

The earliest written records of yoga philosophy are found in the texts of Patanjali's Yoga Sutras, which outline the eight limbs of yoga. These include:

Yama: moral guidelines for living a virtuous life, such as non-violence, truthfulness, and non-stealing.

Niyama: self-discipline and personal practices, such as cleanliness, contentment, and self-study.

Asana: physical postures to purify the body and promote physical and mental well-being.

Pranayama: breath control to purify and balance the energy in the body.

Pratyahara: withdrawal of the senses to quiet the mind.

Dharana: concentration to focus the mind.

Dhyana: meditation to achieve a state of inner peace and insight.

Samadhi: enlightenment, or union with the universal self.

Yoga philosophy also includes the belief in the importance of living a balanced and healthy lifestyle, including proper diet and natural remedies, and the cultivation of inner peace and self-realization.

It is also important to note that Yoga is not just a physical practice but also a spiritual one and it encourages the development of a healthy and balanced lifestyle, with emphasis on proper diet and the use of natural remedies.

Yoga philosophy is open to interpretation and can be practiced in many different ways. It is an individual practice, and each person's journey is unique, but the ultimate goal is the same: to achieve a state of inner peace and enlightenment.

**The 8 limbs of yoga**

The 8 limbs of yoga, also known as Ashtanga Yoga, are a systematic approach to the practice of yoga that was outlined in the Yoga Sutras of Patanjali. These 8 limbs serve as a roadmap for spiritual growth and self-discipline, leading to the ultimate goal of achieving enlightenment or liberation (moksha). The 8 limbs are:

Yama: ethical guidelines for living a virtuous life, such as non-violence, truthfulness, non-stealing, non-possessiveness and continence.

Niyama: personal disciplines and observances, such as cleanliness, contentment, self-study, self-surrender, and devotion to the divine.

Asana: physical postures that help to purify the body and promote physical and mental well-being.

Pranayama: breath control to purify and balance the energy in the body.

Pratyahara: withdrawal of the senses to quiet the mind.

Dharana: concentration to focus the mind.

Dhyana: meditation to achieve a state of inner peace and insight.

Samadhi: enlightenment, or union with the universal self.

It is important to note that these 8 limbs are not meant to be followed in a linear fashion, but rather as a holistic approach to the practice of yoga, each limb supports and informs the others.

Yama and niyama, the first two limbs, lays the foundation for ethical and moral principles, creating a stable and harmonious environment for the practice of the following limbs. Asana, pranayama and pratyahara, the next three limbs, focus on purifying the body and mind. Dharana, dhyana, and samadhi, the final three limbs, focus on concentration, meditation, and enlightenment.

Practicing all 8 limbs of yoga can help to promote physical and mental well-being, increase self-awareness and self-discipline, and ultimately lead to the ultimate goal of achieving enlightenment or liberation.

**How philosophy can enhance your yoga practice**

Incorporating the philosophy of yoga into your practice can enhance your experience in several ways:

It can provide a deeper understanding of the purpose and meaning of the practice. Knowing the history and purpose of the postures, breathing techniques and other practices, can give you a more profound understanding of what you are doing, and why.

It can help to align your practice with your values and beliefs. Understanding the ethical principles of yoga, such as non-violence and truthfulness, can help you to align your practice with your personal values and beliefs, making it more meaningful and fulfilling.

It can help to develop a more holistic practice. Yoga is not just a physical practice, but also a spiritual and mental one. Incorporating the philosophy of yoga can help to develop a more holistic practice that addresses the needs of the body, mind, and spirit.

It can help to cultivate self-awareness. Yoga philosophy encourages self-study, introspection, and self-reflection, which can help to increase self-awareness and understanding of one's own mind and emotions.

It can help to develop a non-judgmental attitude. Yoga philosophy emphasizes the importance of non-attachment and equanimity, which can help to develop a non-judgmental attitude towards oneself and others.

It can help to develop a sense of discipline. The principles of yoga philosophy, such as self-discipline and self-study, can help to develop a sense of discipline that can be beneficial in other areas of your life.

It can help to develop a sense of purpose. Yoga philosophy provides a sense of purpose and direction for the practice, helping you to stay motivated and focused on your goals.

It can help to promote inner peace and self-realization. Yoga philosophy aims to cultivate inner peace, contentment and self-realization, which can lead to a greater sense of well-being and fulfillment in life.

By incorporating the philosophy of yoga into your practice, you can gain a deeper understanding of the practice and its purpose, align your practice with your values, and develop a more holistic, self-aware, and fulfilling practice.

# Conclusion

In conclusion, incorporating the philosophy of yoga into your practice can greatly enhance your experience. By understanding the history, purpose, and principles of yoga, you can align your practice with your values and beliefs, gain a deeper understanding of the practice and its purpose, and develop a more holistic, self-aware, and fulfilling practice. The 8 limbs of yoga serve as a roadmap for spiritual growth and self-discipline, providing guidance for both physical and mental practice. Incorporating the principles of yama and niyama, asana, pranayama, pratyahara, dharana, dhyana, and samadhi can help to purify the body and mind, increase self-awareness and self-discipline, and ultimately lead to the ultimate goal of achieving enlightenment or liberation. Remember that yoga is an individual practice, and each person's journey is unique. The key is to have patience and consistency, listen to your body and honor its limitations, and remember that yoga is not a competition, but rather a path to self-discovery and inner peace.

Printed by Libri Plureos GmbH in Hamburg,
Germany